Race First Aid

A Pocket Manual with Management Pearls

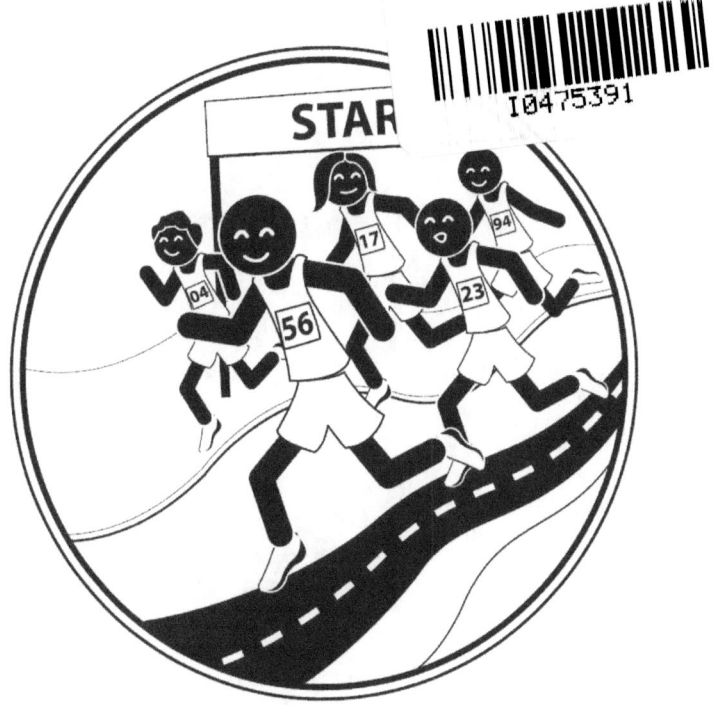

Jeremy Joslin, MD

ACKNOWLEDGMENTS

To my department colleagues in Emergency Medicine at SUNY Upstate Medical Center who support my interest in advancing the science of race medicine and the safety of the endurance athlete and to my wife who supports my academic pursuits despite many days away from home,
I am exceptionally grateful.

CONTRIBUTORS

Two of the brightest and most motivated medical students I've met have invested their efforts into this book's content and mission:

Dylan Kellogg
Nathaniel Herr

Edited by Robert Worthing, MD
Illustrated by Travis Bruce
Cover photo by Glen Delman Photography
www.glendelman.com

ISBN: 978-1460993699

CONTENTS

FORWARD

Race First Aid is like no other first aid manual.

First, we've formatted it to include information specific to your particular role in the race. If you're a general volunteer, you might not want to wade through volumes of dense medical information. Likewise, if you're a medical volunteer, you want to know what you should be doing right now for the patient in front of you, even if you're not a physician, and even if you don't have a diagnosis in mind.

Second, we've tried to really condense the information presented down to the essentials of what you might encounter during a race. While many first aid manuals cover many of these topics quite nicely, we really wanted to be comprehensive in race-specific problems while removing all the non-race-specific problems that are likely to just result in a heavier book and more difficult job of locating a given problem expediently.

You'll notice that we are inclusive of both traditional road races and the circumstances of a remote, expedition-length race. And while the format may take a few reads to get used to, we hope you will become facile with it and come to enjoy using it. Your feedback is always welcome should you be so inclined to provide it. Please contact the author at jeremy.joslin@gmail.com with your comments.

Please remember that this book's advice should never replace that of a licensed and trained medical provider who is on-scene and responsible for the patient.

1.) HEAT-RELATED ILLNESS
Dylan Kellogg

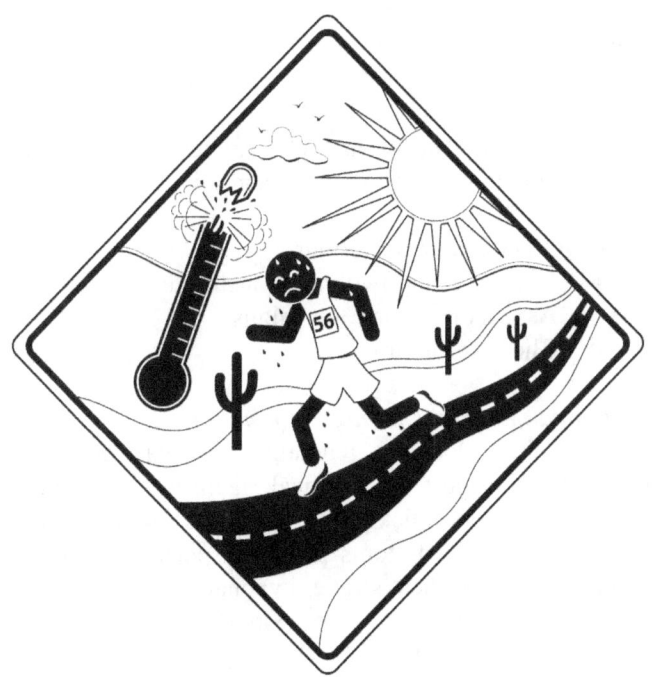

Heat-Related Illness

Collapse (Exercise Associated Collapse)

Explanation: A brief loss of consciousness in an active athlete.

Medical Definition: AKA heat syncope. Brief syncopal episode due to diminished preload resulting from peripheral vasodilation and venous pooling.

Signs & Symptoms: Syncope, dizziness, orthostatic hypotension that occur immediately after cessation of activity or after prolonged standing in the heat.

General Volunteer Instructions:
- Have athlete lie down in a cool area.
- Elevate legs.
- Provide fluid with electrolytes (sports drink) if athlete is fully conscious and thirsty.

Medical Personnel Instructions:
- Review general volunteer instructions.
- Assess orthostatic vital signs.
- Check for injuries.

Additional Medical Director Information:
This condition does not generally necessitate evacuation or emergent transport to medical facilities. Resolution of symptoms occurs quickly and may be considered sufficient for re-entry. If symptoms persist (especially mental status changes), rule out heat stroke, hyponatremia, or alternatives. Bystanders can experience syncope from standing for long periods in the heat due to similar physiology of pooling and

Heat-Related Illness

venodilation.

(Portions of Recommendations Adapted from: Forgey, 63; Noakes)

Heat-Related Illness

Heat Rash

Explanation: Rash that occurs in a hot, humid environment.

Medical Definition: AKA milaria rubra. The rash is caused by blocking of sweat glands.

Signs & Symptoms: Itchy rash of tiny red or white bumps.

General Volunteer Instructions:
- Remove athlete from hot environment.
- Remove any wet clothing.
- Dry the skin.

Medical Personnel Instructions:
- Review general volunteer instructions.
- Provide symptomatic treatment.
- Prevention is the best management.

Additional Medical Director Information:
This condition does not generally necessitate evacuation or emergent transport to medical facilities. Some rashes may resolve shortly after cooling and drying skin, while the remainder typically resolve in 7-10 days. Prolonged or repeated cases of heat rash may, on a rare occasion, lead to a secondary bacterial infection which may necessitate non-emergent evacuation if not manageable with antibiotic treatment.

(Portions of Recommendations Adapted from: Seto)

Heat-Related Illness

Heat Cramps

Explanation: Cramping of active muscles in a hot environment.

Medical Definition: AKA heat tetany. Muscle cramping due to electrolyte imbalance, volume depletion, hyperventilation, respiratory alkalosis, etc.

Signs & Symptoms: Painful contraction of muscles.

General Volunteer Instructions:
- Remove from hot environment.
- Encourage athlete to rest.
- Provide fluid with electrolytes (sports drink).
- Encourage gentle stretching of cramped muscles.

Medical Personnel Instructions:
- Review general volunteer instructions.
- Encourage athletes who have a history of developing cramps to increase their salt intake and drink when thirsty.

Additional Medical Director Information:
Cases of heat cramps may range from carpopedal cramping to contraction of large muscle groups such as the abdominal muscles. This condition does not generally necessitate evacuation or emergent transport to medical facilities, and resolution of symptoms may be considered sufficient for re-entry. If symptoms recur, consider having the athlete rest for 24-hours.

Heat-Related Illness

Sodium depletion is usually implicated in research studies, as opposed to the common perception of potassium depletion as the etiology. An alternative hypothesis is that cramping may develop as a result of a hyperosmolar state secondary to volume depletion. In either case, fluid with electrolytes should be beneficial. Since respiratory alkalosis has also been implicated, encouraging an athlete to breath into a paper bag may also reduce the cramping.

(Portions of Recommendations Adapted from: Carline, 117; Forgey, 63; Seto)

Heat-Related Illness

Heat Edema

Explanation: Accumulation of fluid in hands and feet.

Medical Definition: Vasodilation and interstitial edema in peripheral extremities.

Signs & Symptoms: Swollen hands and feet.

General Volunteer Instructions:
- Have athlete rest in cool area.
- Elevate swollen limbs.

Medical Personnel Instructions:
- Review general volunteer instructions.
- Evaluate for any other abnormal signs or symptoms which indicate a process other than this benign condition.

Additional Medical Director Information:
This condition does not generally necessitate evacuation or emergent transport to medical facilities, and resolution of symptoms may be considered sufficient for re-entry, as the condition is usually indicative of incomplete acclimatization.

(Portions of Recommendations Adapted from: Seto)

Heat-Related Illness

Heat Exhaustion

Explanation: Body is producing more heat than it is losing. This causes fatigue and a general unwell feeling. It is one of the most common heat illnesses.

Medical Definition: Thermoregulatory dysfunction with an elevated core temperature. **Because the exact defining temperature differs by text, we do not condone using temperature to define this illness**.

Signs & Symptoms: Weakness, inability to exercise, headache, nausea, faintness, anorexia, dyspnea, tachycardia, normal BP. Skin can be warm or cool, and is usually sweaty. The presence of sweat does not exclude heat stroke (a common misconception).

General Volunteer Instructions:
- Rest athlete in cool area.
- Administer fluid with electrolytes (sports drink).
- Initiate cooling with wet towels and fanning.

Medical Personnel Instructions:
- Review general volunteer instructions.
- Assess athlete for signs and symptoms of heat stroke.
- Review *Heat Stroke* section for more information. This is one of the most important differentiations in race medicine.

Additional Medical Director Information:
This condition does not generally necessitate evacuation or emergent transport to medical facilities, and resolution of

Heat-Related Illness

symptoms may be considered sufficient for re-entry - this may take up to 24 hours. True alteration in mental status indicates heat stroke and should be aggressively treated as such.

(Portions of Recommendations Adapted from: Carline, 117-118; Forgey, 63-64; Seto)

Heat-Related Illness

Heat Stroke

Explanation: The body has lost the ability to cool itself. This is a serious medical condition that can result in **permanent organ system damage or death** if not recognized and treated rapidly.

Medical Definition: Thermoregulatory dysfunction with an elevated core temperature. **Because the exact defining temperature differs by text, we do not condone using temperature to define this illness.**

Signs & Symptoms: An altered mental status ranging from simple confusion or bizarre behavior to complete unresponsiveness. Ataxia, a difficulty with coordinating movements such as walking, is commonly seen and should be a major red flag. An example is a wobbly run, or inability to move in a straight line. Skin is typically flushed, hot, and sweaty (but may appear dry).

General Volunteer Instructions:
- Contact Medical Personnel Instructions immediately with ANY suspicion of this illness.
- Have athlete rest in a cool area.
- Remove athlete's clothing.
- Initiate aggressive cooling with wetting of skin and fanning.
- If available place ice packs or ice-water soaked towels against neck, armpits, and groin.
- High pulse and breathing rate with low blood pressure may occur.

Heat-Related Illness

- Note: symptoms may improve with rest, but this does not obviate the need for definitive treatment and medical intervention.

Medical Personnel Instructions:
- Review general volunteer instructions.
- **Prepare for immediate evacuation or transport**.
- Implement rapid cooling measures as soon as possible.
- Obtain rectal temperature, but do not base diagnosis on this since body temperature may have cooled in the interim and does not negate the possibly higher temperature present before formal measurement.
- Do not give antipyretics since this condition is not caused by hypothylamic set point elevation or fever.
- Consider cold water immersion or serial body wraps with ice-water soaked sheets (taco or burrito cooling method) while awaiting medical director.
- Monitor ABC's.
- Initiate intravenous fluids according to protocol, equipment availability, and scope of practice.
- Discontinue cooling when rectal temperature = 39°C (102°F) to avoid reflex hypothermia or overcooling.

Additional Medical Director Information:
This condition represents a true medical emergency and current guidelines recommend immediate evacuation or emergent transport to medical facilities and formal evaluation. Use caution with individuals who have previous history of heat stroke when considering event entry. Consider close communication with accepting medical facility to decrease time to cooling, and to relay the gravity of the condition.

Heat-Related Illness

We recommend aggressive cooling initiated in the field before transport.

(Portions of Recommendations Adapted from: Carline, 118-119; Forgey, 64; Seto)

Heat-Related Illness

Hyponatremia

Explanation: Less than the normal amount of salt dissolved in the bloodstream likely from drinking too much regular water.

Medical Definition: Low serum sodium concentration. While the condition can be due to diminished salt intake or increased salt excretion, in athletes it is generally due to having a greater fluid intake (through drinking) than loss (through sweat and urine). The problem is exacerbated by increased arginine vasopressin secretion in response to exertion. Use of non-steroidal anti-inflammatory drugs such as ibuprofen also contributes to the pathophysiology.

Signs & Symptoms: Nausea, vomiting headache, confusion, disorientation, seizures, coma.

General Volunteer Instructions:
- Encourage athlete to drink only if thirsty (not as much as possible).
- Provide fluid with electrolytes (sports drink).
- Avoid plain water during extended races.

Medical Personnel Instructions:
- Review general volunteer instructions.
- Because symptoms are very similar to heat illness, it is important to get a sense of the athlete's fluid intake (Water or sports drink? How much? How often?).
- The best treatment is prevention. Encourage athletes to drink only when thirsty and to consume sports drinks or salty snacks rather than water alone.

Heat-Related Illness

Additional Medical Director Information:
Point of care electrolyte testing is suggested to define the degree of derangement. In the presence of altered mental status or seizure, consider a bolus of hypertonic (3%) saline solution. Evacuation or emergent transport to medical facilities is suggested for even minor cases due to propensity to worsen without close care. Normal saline will worsen exercise associated hyponatremia due to naturesis which occurs more rapidly than aquaresis.

(Portions of Recommendations Adapted from: Forgey, 73-76; Noakes; Rogers)

2.) COLD-RELATED ILLNESS
Dylan Kellogg

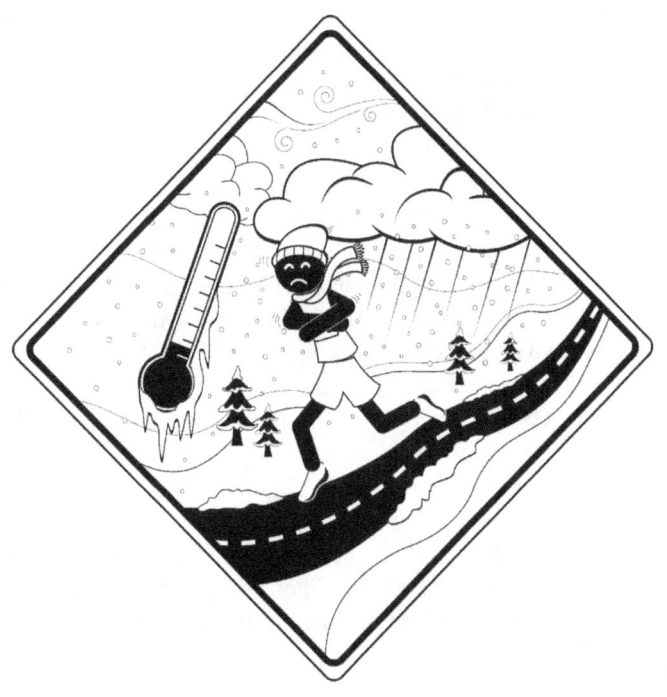

Cold-Related Illness

Frostbite

Explanation: Body part is frozen.

Medical Definition: Localized tissue injury or death due to damage caused by the freezing of cells and tissue.

Signs & Symptoms: Skin may be discolored (white or blue) and firm. Coldness, numbness, or loss of sensation in affected area.

General Volunteer Instructions:
- Do not attempt to rewarm (or rub) the frozen part as this may worsen the injury.
- Contact Medical Personnel immediately.
- Provide athlete with food and water and protect from further injury.

Medical Personnel Instructions:
- Review general volunteer instructions.
- Document appearance of injury, paying attention to blisters, color of skin, any woody hardness, waxiness, etc.
- If refreezing cannot be prevented, do not rewarm.
- Assess and treat for hypothermia prior to initiating rewarming.

Additional Medical Director Information:
Time to treatment does not significantly impact outcome under many circumstances. Therefore, address all variables when considering rapid rewarming in the field.

Cold-Related Illness

If feet are affected, do not rewarm prior to evacuation. Debilitating pain and dysthesias are common during and after rewarming (and may complicate evacuation), necessitating adequate pain relief measures. If field rewarming is considered, immerse injured extremity in 40-42°C (104-108°F) water bath for 15-30 minutes or until thawed. Loosely splint the affected extremity. Ibuprofen or a similar NSAID should be administered both to assist in pain control and minimize tissue damage from inflammation. Narcotic pain medication should be used for further pain control as prehospital facilities and scope of practice allow. Ensure adequate hydration.

Current guidelines recommend evacuation or transport to medical facilities and formal evaluation prior to re-entry. Immediacy of the evacuation or transport is at the race director's discretion and should depend on the severity of the condition.

(Portions of Recommendations Adapted from: Forgey, 60-61; Seto)

Cold-Related Illness

Immersion Foot

Explanation: Continued exposure to cold and moist environment (such as continuously wearing wet shoes and socks) damages the skin.

Medical Definition: AKA trench foot. While the pathophysiology is not completely understood, injury to soft tissue results from prolonged exposure to cool temperature above freezing. Time to development is variable, but typically more than one day of exposure is thought to be necessary. If untreated, it can progress to gangrene.

Signs & Symptoms: Cold, swollen foot with mottled skin. This progresses to erythema and blisters, and finally to pallor or cyanosis. Numbness is common initially, and progresses to aches, pain, and infections. Peripheral pulses may be diminished.

General Volunteer Instructions:
- Carefully remove cold and wet clothing and replace with warm and dry items.
- Provide fluid with electrolytes (sports drink).

Medical Personnel Instructions:
- Review general volunteer instructions.
- Document appearance of injury and make special note of areas of infection or gangrene.
- Administer ibuprofen for pain.
- The best treatment is prevention. Athletes should be encouraged to change socks regularly and keep feet dry.

Cold-Related Illness

Additional Medical Director Information:
Current guidelines recommend evacuation or emergent transport to medical facilities and formal evaluation prior to re-entry. Race directors may wish to consider immediate evacuation or emergent transport and should consider that an injured foot may be too painful to allow for a walking evacuation.

(Portions of Recommendations Adapted from: Castellani; Isaac 157-158; Forgey, 61)

Cold-Related Illness

Mild Hypothermia

Explanation: Body's heat production is less than heat loss, but patient is attempting to compensate (e.g. by shivering).

Medical Definition: Thermoregulatory dysfunction with a core temperature between 32°C (90°F) and 35°C (95°F). Be aware that hypothermia may develop in athletes immediately post-race.

Signs & Symptoms: Shivering, loss of judgment & fine motor control, slurred speech, ataxia, cold extremities, pale & cool skin, increased urination (cold diuresis).

General Volunteer Instructions:
- Initiate warming of the athlete while changing out any wet clothing.
- Protect from further heat loss.
- Provide warm, high energy food and beverages such as those with high sugar content.
- If possible, apply external heat sources to chest and armpits, but do not place directly against skin.

Medical Personnel Instructions:
- Review general volunteer instructions.
- Asses vital signs.
- Confirm athlete is in positive thermoregulation (that they are warming and preferably shivering).
- Confirm that judgment and coordination are intact.
- If mental status is altered, reconsider the diagnosis or severity of hypothermia.

Cold-Related Illness

Additional Medical Director Information:
With careful evaluation, this condition does not generally necessitate evacuation or emergent transport to medical facilities, and resolution of symptoms may be considered sufficient for re-entry. Ensure implementation of adequate measures by the racer to prevent recurrence.

(Portions of Recommendations Adapted from: Forgey, 55-56; Seto)

Cold-Related Illness

Severe hypothermia

Explanation: The body's ability to compensate for continued heat loss is overwhelmed (i.e. no shivering).

Medical Definition: Thermoregulatory dysfunction with a core temperature < 32°C (90°F).

Signs & Symptoms: Altered mental status, loss of coordination, decreased level of consciousness, fixed & dilated pupils, and hypotension. Heart and respiratory rates may be undetectable. Athlete may no longer be shivering.

General Volunteer Instructions:
- Contact Medical Personnel immediately if severe hypothermia is suspected.
- Handle athlete gently, moving as little as possible. Jolting movements or chest wall agitation can cause heart rhythm problems.
- Remove wet clothes and insulate with warm, dry clothes.
- Protect from further heat loss.
- Apply external heat to chest and armpits but do not place directly on the skin.

Medical Personnel Instructions:
- Review general volunteer instructions.
- Assess heart rate (at carotid pulse) and respiratory rates for one minute each.
- If no pulse or respirations are detected after one minute you may provide positive pressure ventilation.
- Protect the patient from additional heat loss.

Cold-Related Illness

Additional Medical Director Information:
This condition represents a true medical emergency and current guidelines recommend immediate evacuation or emergent transport to medical facilities, and formal evaluation prior to re-entry.

This can be a difficult condition to manage without electric cardiac monitoring. Be cognizant of the fact that a severely hypothermic patient may be able to maintain metabolic demands with a profoundly depressed cardiac rate. This peculiar situation of physiologic preservation can actually be upset by initiation of CPR as thoracic compressions may convert a perfusing bradycardia into a non-perfusing dysrhythmia such as ventricular fibrillation.

(Portions of Recommendations Adapted from: Forgey, 55-57; Seto)

3.) ENVIRONMENTAL INJURIES
Dylan Kellogg

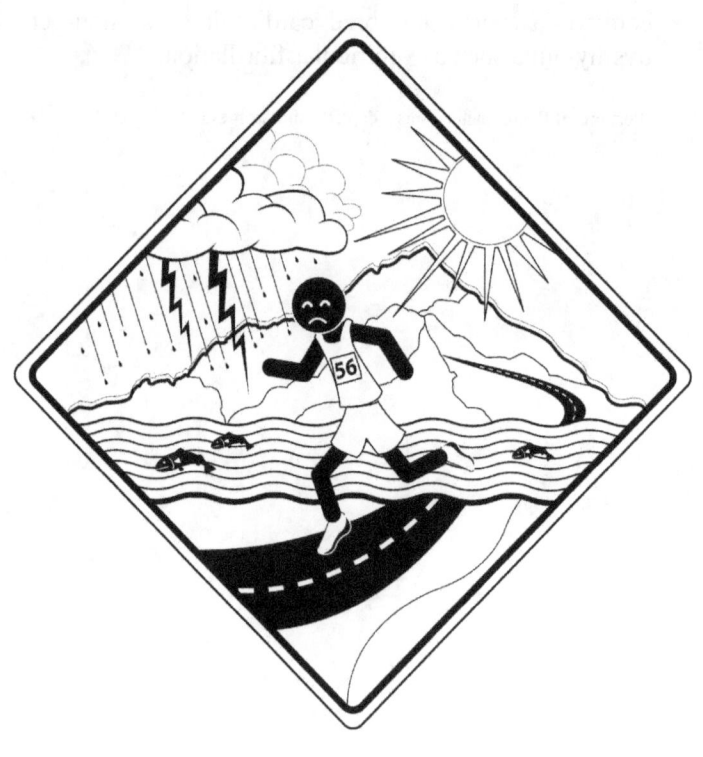

Environmental Injuries

Sunburn

Explanation: Prolonged exposure to sunlight damages exposed skin causing painful burns.

Medical Definition: Erythema with or without blistering resulting from UV-triggered cell death, dilation of dermal blood vessels, and inflammatory response.

Signs & Symptoms: Skin is red, warm and painful; blisters may be present if severe.

General Volunteer Instructions:
- Cover burn to keep out of sun.
- If in a warm environment, consider cooling skin with water.

Medical Personnel Instructions:
- Review general volunteer instructions.
- Prevent further damage from sun and apply a sterile dressing.
- Attempt to keep blisters intact for as long as possible, or manage them by puncturing them in a controlled environment that can remain sterile after draining.
- Consider ibuprofen for pain.
- A mild topical anti-inflammatory such as aloe may be used.
- Encourage future sunscreen use.

Additional Medical Director Information:
This condition does not generally necessitate evacuation or emergent transport to medical facilities. Relief of symptoms

Environmental Injuries

and implementation of prevention measures may be considered sufficient for re-entry.

(Portions of Recommendations Adapted from: Forgey, 26-27; Seto)

Environmental Injuries

Altitude Sickness (Acute Mountain Sickness—AMS)

Explanation: The brain is not getting enough oxygen because of thinner atmosphere at high altitude.

Medical Definition: A syndrome resulting from tissue hypoxia due to decreased partial pressure of oxygen at altitude.

Signs & Symptoms: The most common initial symptom is headache, but other early symptoms can include anorexia, nausea, vomiting, dizziness, lightheadedness, sleep disturbances, and lethargy. Alarming late stage manifestations are High Altitude Cerebral Edema (HACE), which initially presents with ataxia and mental status changes, and may progress to catastrophic brain herniation; and High Altitude Pulmonary Edema (HAPE), which presents with dry cough, rales and decreased exercise tolerance, and progresses to pink or bloody sputum and respiratory distress.

General Volunteer Instructions:
- Have athlete rest and contact Medical Personnel.
- Monitor for abnormal behavior, and protect from falls or other possible mechanisms of self-injury resulting from loss of coordination or mental capacity.
- Do not leave athlete unattended.

Medical Personnel Instructions:
- Review general volunteer instructions.
- Insist on the athlete resting if in a safe environment.
- Administer supplemental O_2 if available.

Environmental Injuries

- Descend if symptoms do not resolve or are severe.
- Ibuprofen (400-600mg) or acetaminophen (1000mg) may be given for headache pain.
- Any anti-emetic medication can be used for nausea if included in your protocol and scope of practice.
- The best treatment of AMS is descent. However, if rescue pharmacotherapy is needed while planning or effecting descent, consider acetazolamide or dexamethasone.

Additional Medical Director Information:
If symptoms do not resolve with descent, evacuation or emergent transport to definitive care may be warranted. Otherwise, clinical judgment dictates when an athlete may resume activity. When in doubt, consult with an expert in altitude illness.

(Portions of Recommendations Adapted from: Forgey, 49-50, Seto)

Environmental Injuries

Lightning Strike

Explanation: Injury due to lightning strike.

Medical Definition: A broad spectrum of injury dependant on strike subtype, the path of current through the body, and other factors.

Signs & Symptoms: Can be quite variable ranging from minimal orthopedic injuries or burns to seizures, spinal injuries, unresponsiveness, and cardiopulmonary arrest. Lightning can cause arrhythmia if cardiac tissue is affected, or respiratory arrest if central nervous tissue is affected.

General Volunteer Instructions:
- Ensure scene safety (threat of additional nearby strike).
- Determine number of injured people.
- Begin CPR on any athlete who is not breathing.
- Contact Medical Personnel.

Medical Personnel Instructions:
- Review general volunteer instructions.
- Assess and treat ABC's as necessary.
- Assess for burns and other injuries that may not be immediately obvious. Treat as indicated.
- Remember that a patient who requires CPR may convert to a perfusing rhythm before their medulla can re-initiate spontaneous respirations.
- Be prepared to continue providing artificial respirations even in a patient with adequate cardiac activity.

Environmental Injuries

Additional Medical Director Information:
This condition represents a true medical emergency and current guidelines recommend immediate evacuation or emergent transport to medical facilities and formal evaluation prior to re-entry. Clinical judgment regarding expediency of evacuation may be used in cases of indirect exposure to lightning when the athlete does not exhibit any evidence of injury or illness.

(Portions of Recommendations Adapted from: Forgey, 65-66)

Environmental Injuries

Immersion Injury

Explanation: Injury due to water inhalation or laryngospasm.

Medical Definition: Two mechanisms are classically described in drowning and immersion injuries. In the first, inhalation of water results in an inability of gas exchange to occur in the alveoli. In the second, airway spasm (secondary to water exposure) prevents both air and water from reaching the alveoli.

Signs & Symptoms: Unresponsiveness, lack of breathing, coughing, vomiting.

General Volunteer Instructions:
- Remove athlete from water without compromising the safety of rescuers.
- Begin CPR if patient is not breathing or if unresponsive.
- Contact Medical Personnel.

Medical Personnel Instructions:
- Review general volunteer instructions.
- Assess and treat ABC's as necessary.
- Monitor for development of respiratory distress.
- Evaluate for presence of concomitant immersion injury such as hypothermia, and treat appropriately.
- If in a remote location, your medical director may consider terminating CPR if the patient is not resuscitated after 30 minutes.

Environmental Injuries

Additional Medical Director Information:
This condition represents a true medical emergency and current guidelines recommend immediate evacuation or emergent transport to medical facilities and formal evaluation prior to re-entry. Closely observe all patients during evacuation or transport for development of delayed respiratory insult which may occur several hours after submersion. Current literature suggests much of the previously assumed pathophysiology in this disease process may be incorrect.

(Portions of Recommendations Adapted from: Forgey 13-14; Isaac, 160)

4.) ORTHOPEDIC INJURIES
Nathaniel Herr

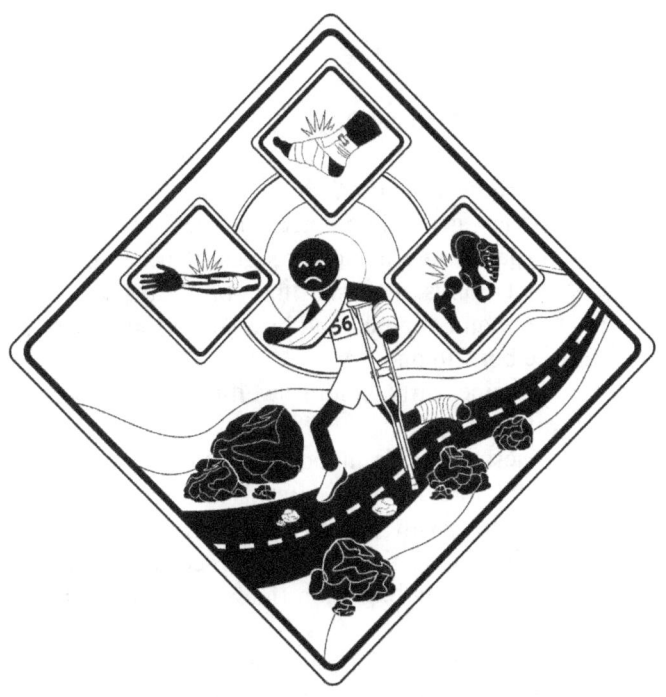

Orthopedic Injuries

Suspected Fracture

Explanation: Broken Bone.

Medical Definition: Fracture.

Signs & Symptoms: Pain, tenderness, swelling, discoloration, deformity, guarding, crepitus, point tenderness, rigidity, and diminished use of injured limb.

General Volunteer Instructions:
- Have athlete rest and quickly assess for other injuries.
- Try to immobilize the limb, or reduce the need to move it.
- Contact Medical Personnel.

Medical Personnel Instructions:
- Review general volunteer instructions.
- Inspect and palpate for signs of fracture by feeling for crepitus, assessing the ability to use the injured limb, and appreciating how much the patient guards the bone in question.
- Examine early before swelling makes examination difficult.
- Assess distal circulation, sensation, and movement.
- If fracture is open, treat as a high risk wound by cleaning with copious amounts of potable water. Reduce if within protocol and scope of practice.
- Apply immobilization including joint above and below.
- Use ibuprofen for pain unless prehospital facilities and scope of practice allow for narcotic use.

Orthopedic Injuries

Additional Medical Director Information:
Current guidelines recommend evacuation or emergent transport to medical facilities and formal evaluation prior to re-entry, although urgency of evacuation should be dictated by severity and consequences of the injury. Consider immediate evacuation if the fracture is open or associated with significant hemorrhage or if cardiovascular or neurologic compromise is present.

(Portions of Recommendations Adapted from: Forgey, 29-32)

Orthopedic Injuries

Suspected Sprain or Strain

Explanation: Pulled muscle, twisted ankle, etc.

Medical Definition: Injury to muscle, ligament or tendon resulting from movement through the limits of range of motion.

Signs & Symptoms: Pain, tenderness, swelling, and bruising.

General Volunteer Instructions:
- Have athlete rest and quickly assess for other injuries.
- Try to immobilize the limb, or reduce the need to move it.
- Contact Medical Personnel.

Medical Personnel Instructions:
- Review general volunteer instructions.
- Inspect and palpate for signs of fracture by feeling for crepitus, assessing the ability to use the injured limb, and appreciating how much the patient guards the bone in question.
- Examine early before swelling makes examination difficult.
- Assess for weight bearing, range of motion, joint stability, and strength.
- **Protect** extremity by splinting.
- **Rest** the extremity.
- Apply cold therapy without placing **ice** directly on skin.
- Apply **compression** using an ACE wrap or similar bandage.

Orthopedic Injuries

- Utilize **elevation** to reduce swelling.
- Use ibuprofen for pain.

Additional Medical Director Information:
Current guidelines recommend evacuation or emergent transport to medical facilities and formal evaluation prior to re-entry.

(Portions of Recommendations Adapted from: Trojian)

Orthopedic Injuries

Suspected Dislocation

Explanation: Bone has come out of joint.

Medical Definition: Disruption of proper bony articulation within a joint.

Signs & Symptoms: Restricted range of motion, deformity, pain, swelling, and bruising.

General Volunteer Instructions:
- Have athlete rest and quickly assess for other injuries.
- Try to immobilize the limb, or reduce the need to move it.
- Contact Medical Personnel.

Medical Personnel Instructions:
- Review general volunteer instructions.
- Evaluate for concurrent fracture as described under *Suspected Fracture.*
- Assess for deformity, compromise of distal circulation, sensation, and distal movement.
- If no fractures are suspected, and if within your scope of practice, consider reduction followed by reassessment of distal circulation, sensation and motion.
- Splint and immobilize.
- Use ibuprofen for pain.

Additional Medical Director Information: Current guidelines recommend evacuation or emergent transport to medical facilities and formal evaluation prior to re-entry. Medical

Orthopedic Injuries

directors may wish to consider immediate evacuation if the joint cannot be reduced or if there is neurological or vascular compromise.

(Portions of Recommendations Adapted from: Forgey, 32-35)

5.) SOFT TISSUE INJURIES
Nathaniel Herr

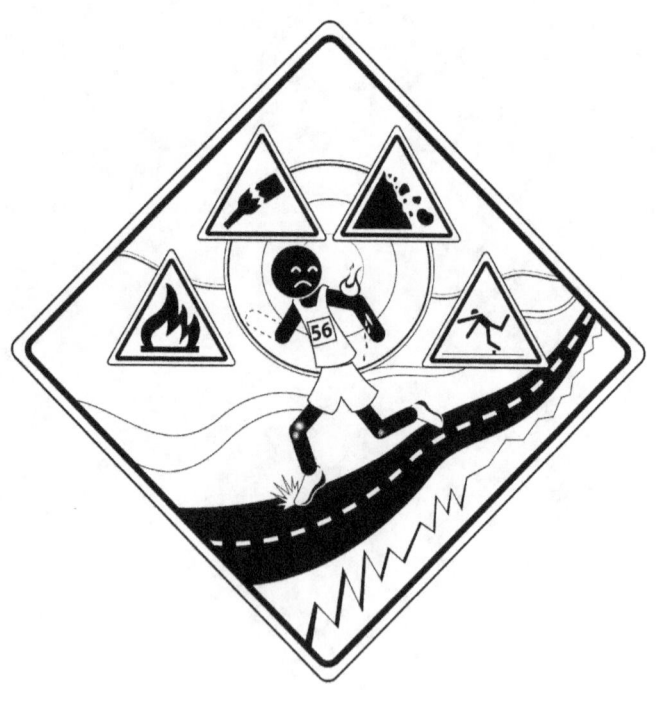

Soft Tissue Injuries

Contusion

Explanation: A bruise.

Medical Definition: Tissue hematoma.

Signs & Symptoms: Pain, induration, discoloration of skin.

General Volunteer Instructions:
- Have athlete rest and quickly assess for other injuries.
- Contact Medical Personnel.

Medical Personnel Instructions:
- Review general volunteer instructions.
- Evaluate for other associated injury such as fractures as described under *Suspected Fracture.*
- Splint for comfort and protection.
- Once swelling is controlled (usually 72 hours), consider heat.

Additional Medical Director Information:
This condition does not generally necessitate evacuation or emergent transport to medical facilities as clinical judgment of the severity of injury and the likelihood of concomitant occult fractures can be used to determine whether the athlete may continue to participate.

(Portions of Recommendations Adapted from: Forgey, 21)

Soft Tissue Injuries

Black Nail

Explanation: Blood blister beneath toenail or fingernail.

Medical Definition: Subungal hematoma.

Signs & Symptoms: Pain, pressure, and discoloration of nail.

General Volunteer Instructions:
- Have athlete rest and quickly assess for other injuries.
- Contact Medical Personnel or allow athlete to manage on their own if comfortable and experienced.

Medical Personnel Instructions:
- Review general volunteer instructions.
- Painful subungual hematomas involving greater than 25% of the nail can be decompressed using a sharp sterile blade, hypodermic needle, or hot paperclip to provide relief.
- If you have not practiced this in the past, you should consider consultation with someone with experience since it is a potentially painful experience if the procedure is performed incorrectly.
- Re-accumulation of blood can be drained through original hole after re-instrumentation.

Additional Medical Director Information:
This condition does not generally necessitate evacuation or emergent transport to medical facilities, and resolution of symptoms or decision of athlete may be considered sufficient for re-entry.
(Portions of Recommendations Adapted from: Forgey, 21; Micheli, 177)

Soft Tissue Injuries

Abrasion

Explanation: A scrape.

Medical Definition: Wound with minimal bleeding limited to the epidermis.

Signs & Symptoms: Pain, induration, redness, inflammation, minimal bleeding.

General Volunteer Instructions:
- Have athlete rest and quickly assess for other injuries.
- Apply direct pressure with sterile gauze to stop bleeding.
- Contact Medical Personnel if athlete wishes to be evaluated.

Medical Personnel Instructions:
- Review general volunteer instructions.
- Evaluate underlying structures (bone, muscle, tendons, nerves or blood vessels).
- Clean with a mild soap and water.
- Irrigate with copious amount of clean water which is safe enough to drink.
- Apply thick coating of topical antimicrobial first-aid ointment and dress with sterile gauze.

Additional Medical Director Information:
This condition does not generally necessitate evacuation or emergent transport to medical facilities. Medical directors of multi-day events may wish to consider evacuation if infection or cellulitis develops. Clinical judgment of the

Soft Tissue Injuries

severity of injury can be used to determine whether the athlete may continue to participate.

(Portions of Recommendations Adapted from: Forgey, 21; Micheli, 4)

Soft Tissue Injuries

Laceration or Avulsion

Explanation: A cut.

Medical Definition: Sharp object damaging the dermis.

Signs & Symptoms: Pain, induration, redness, inflammation, bleeding.

General Volunteer Instructions:
- Have athlete rest and quickly assess for other injuries.
- Apply continuous direct pressure with sterile gauze to stop bleeding.
- Contact Medical Personnel.

Medical Personnel Instructions:
- Review general volunteer instructions.
- Evaluate underlying structures (bone, muscle, tendons, nerves or blood vessels).
- Copiously irrigate with water clean enough to drink. Pressure irrigation with a syringe (or plastic bag) is preferred.
- Inspect the wound with sterile forceps and remove debris as needed.
- Dress and bandage the wound with sterile gauze and then apply direct, continuous pressure to control bleeding.
- Continue adding additional gauze and applying pressure until bleeding is controlled.
- For significant bleeding, or obvious arterial bleeding, consider applying two fingers of direct pressure under direct visualization of the bleeding

Soft Tissue Injuries

site to ensure vessel compression. Providing two fingers of direct pressure to terminate bleeding may be more effective than several layers of bulky gauze.

Additional Medical Director Information:
Current guidelines recommend immediate evacuation or emergent transport to medical facilities and formal evaluation prior to re-entry for significant bleeding injuries. Clinical judgment of the severity of injury can be used to determine whether further participation or evacuation is appropriate.

(Portions of Recommendations Adapted from: Forgey, 21-22; Micheli, 4)

Soft Tissue Injuries

Burn

Explanation: Thermal injury.

Medical Definition: Any skin or deep tissue injury from heat, electricity, sun, chemicals, or radiation.

Signs & Symptoms: Pain, induration, redness, inflammation, blistering, charred skin, dehydration, infection.

General Volunteer Instructions:
- Ensure scene safety.
- Stop the burning process.
- Have athlete rest and quickly assess for other injuries.
- Remove all clothing and jewelry from the area immediately surrounding and distal to injury, except where stuck to skin.
- Contact Medical Personnel.

Medical Personnel Instructions:
- Review general volunteer instructions.
- Stop the burning process if not already terminated.
- Gently cover the injury with loose, sterile gauze or burn gel dressing.
- Consider gentle cooling measures for comfort.
- Attempt to keep blisters intact for as long as possible, or manage them by puncturing them in a controlled environment that can remain sterile after draining.
- Ensure adequate hydration and prevent hypothermia.
- If burn has affected the upper body, or if the burn resulted from a flash of fire, you must carefully

consider the potential for airway insult which can lead to swelling of the airway structures and rapidly developing airway compromise.

- The following have been implicated as significant warning signs that airway complications might occur: the presence of hoarse voice, soot in the airway, blackened sputum, singed nasal hairs, and burns to the face.

Additional Medical Director Information:

Current guidelines recommend evacuation or emergent transport to medical facilities and formal evaluation prior to re-entry for significant partial thickness or full thickness burns. Medical directors may wish to consider immediate evacuation if airway injury is suspected or if non-superficial burns total more than 15% of the athlete's total body surface area. The following special categories of burns should be paid due diligence with a low threshold for emergent evacuation: burns to sensitive areas such as the face, hands, feet, or genitals; circumferential burns; and most chemical, electric, or radiation burns.

(Portions of Recommendations Adapted from: Forgey, 24-27; Micheli, 4)

6.) BITES & STINGS
Nathaniel Herr

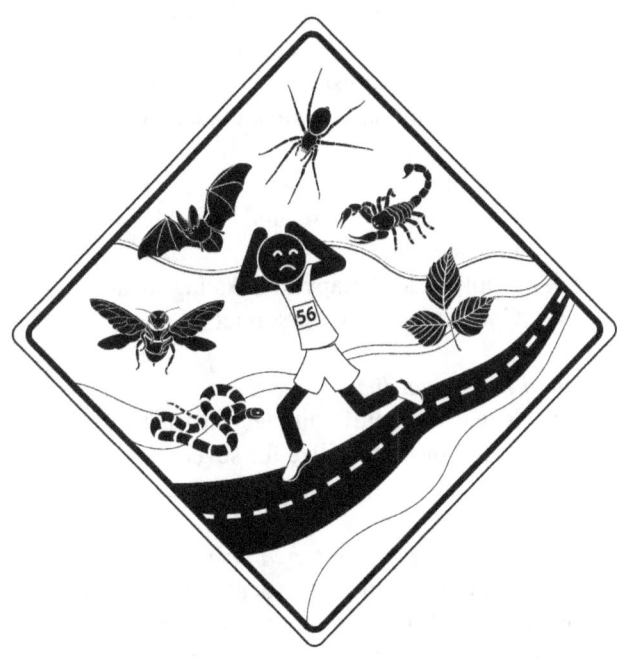

Bites & Stings

Scorpion Sting

Medical Definition: Penetrating wound with envenomation.

Signs & Symptoms: Mild envenomation in which symptoms typically last less than four hours is suggested by pain, minimal swelling, redness, vesicles, tingling, and uncommonly, weakness and numbness.

Severe envenomation is suggested by severe pain, hypersensitivity to touch, pressure, heat and cold, salivation, diaphoresis, perioral paresthesias, dysphagia, gastric distention, hyperactivity, diplopia, nystagmus, visual loss, incontinence, penile erection, exaggerated reflexes, abdominal pain, opisthotonos, seizures, hypertension, hypotension, pulmonary edema, coma, and muscle paralysis.

General Volunteer Instructions:
- Have athlete rest and quickly assess for other injuries.
- Apply cold therapy to the sting location.
- Contact Medical Personnel.

Medical Personnel Instructions:
- Review general volunteer instructions.
- Splint or immobilize for severe pain.
- Administer oral analgesics if needed.

Additional Medical Director Information:
Current guidelines suggest evacuation or emergent transport to medical facilities for severe envenomations (determined by severity of symptoms or body size of athlete). Athletes

Bites & Stings

with only mild symptoms may resume activity based on the clinical judgment of the medical director.

(Portions of Recommendations Adapted from: Forgey, 97-98)

Bites & Stings

Spider Bite

Explanation: In the United States the two most important biting spiders are the black widow and the brown recluse. Bites from these two spiders can result in severe symptoms.

Medical Definition: Penetrating wound with envenomation. Although brown recluse and black widow bites may present with different symptoms and necessitate different definitive treatment, initial first aid for both is the same.

Signs & Symptoms: Redness, pain, and inflammation at the site. For black widow bites: within the first hour, excruciating cramping pain that can be localized or spread to major muscle groups. Hypertension, respiratory distress, seizures and occasionally cardiopulmonary arrest may also develop. For brown recluse bites: within 12 hours a "bull's-eye lesion" centered on a hemorrhagic vesicle may develop and may eventually progress to necrosis. Additionally, nausea, vomiting headache and fever may develop.

General Volunteer Instructions:
- Have athlete rest and quickly assess for other injuries.
- Apply cold to the bite site for comfort.
- Contact Medical Personnel.

Medical Personnel Instructions:
- Review general volunteer instructions.
- Carefully wash the site with clean water.
- Cold packs applied to the bite site may help with pain.
- Offer oral analgesic.

Bites & Stings

- While it may sometimes prove helpful to identify the species in a known spider bite, all spider bites and envenomations can be treated similarly in the field unless species-specific information is readily available.

Additional Medical Director Information:
Current guidelines suggest evacuation or emergent transport to medical facilities for severe symptoms. However, athletes with only mild symptoms can resume activity based on the clinical judgment of the medical director. It should be noted that many skin infections are reflexively blamed on the false presumption of a brown recluse spider bite.

(Portions of Recommendations Adapted from: Forgey, 95-97)

Bites & Stings

Snake Bite - Crotalidae

Explanation: The Crotalidae family, also known as pit vipers, includes rattlesnakes, cottonmouths, and copperheads.

Medical Definition: Penetrating wound with envenomation.

Signs & Symptoms: Redness, pain, inflammation at bite site.

General Volunteer Instructions:
- Have athlete rest and quickly assess for other injuries.
- Contact Medical Personnel.
- Encourage athlete to rest and remain calm.

Medical Personnel Instructions:
- Review general volunteer instructions.
- Mark the borders of swelling to detect spreading. Reassess regularly.
- Gently cleanse the area, apply a sterile dressing and splint the limb.
- Keep extremity at heart level or lower.
- Do not apply pressure dressings, tourniquets or cold to the bite.
- Folk remedies and commercially available products are of no proven benefit and often introduce undo harm.
- If scope of practice and equipment permit, intravenous fluid may be administered to support blood pressure.

Bites & Stings

Additional Medical Director Information:
Current guidelines recommend immediate evacuation or emergent transport to medical facilities and formal evaluation prior to re-entry. If possible, minimize the amount of walking the athlete must do unless walking is required to rapidly evacuate the patient.

(Portions of Recommendations Adapted from: Forgey, 90-93)

Bites & Stings

Snake Bite - Elapidae

Explanation: The Elapidae family includes coral snakes, cobras and sea snakes.

Medical Definition: Penetrating wound with envenomation.

Signs & Symptoms: Initial localized symptoms may be minimal. Systemic symptoms include nausea, vomiting, sweating, myalgias, malaise, paralysis, weakness, blurred vision and respiratory distress. Coagulopathy may develop, resulting in intracerebral hemorrhage with signs and symptoms of increased intracerebral pressure.

General Volunteer Instructions:
- Have athlete rest and quickly assess for other injuries.
- Contact Medical Personnel.
- Encourage athlete to rest and remain calm.

Medical Personnel Instructions:
- Review general volunteer instructions.
- Assume envenomation.
- Apply a compression bandage (as if you were wrapping a sprained ankle) that goes from the bite site, to the top of the limb and back, and then splint the limb.
- Prevent the injured athlete from moving.

Additional Medical Director Information:
Current guidelines recommend immediate evacuation or emergent transport to medical facilities and formal evaluation prior to re-entry. If possible, it is recommended

Bites & Stings

that patients bitten by Elapidae move as little as possible to minimize the likelihood of the venom spreading and the development of systemic symptoms.

(Portions of Recommendations Adapted from: Forgey, 90-93)

Bites & Stings

Bat Bite

Medical Definition: Penetrating wound.

Signs & Symptoms: Redness, pain, or inflammation at the site. Some bat bites do not produce any symptoms or signs of a bite, and bites may go unnoticed.

General Volunteer Instructions:
- Have athlete rest and quickly assess for other injuries.
- Apply cold therapy to the bite site.
- Contact Medical Personnel.

Medical Personnel Instructions:
- Review general volunteer instructions.
- Cleanse wound thoroughly with saline or clean water to reduce viral innoculum.
- Administer rabies immunoglobulin around wound if available.
- Apply antibiotic ointment.
- Do not discount a reported bite because of a lack of visible evidence.

Additional Medical Director Information:
Current guidelines recommend immediate evacuation or emergent transport to medical facilities for hospital evaluation for rabies treatment/prophylaxis with immunoglobulin and vaccination (ideally within 72-hours) prior to re-entry.

(Portions of Recommendations Adapted from: Forgey, 88)

Bites & Stings

Bee Sting

Medical Definition: Penetrating wound, possibly with stinger still embedded. There is a possibility of anaphylactic reaction.

Signs & Symptoms: Localized pain, swelling, and redness. A more serious reaction (anaphylaxis) is indicated by the presence of progressive pruritis, hives, or angioedema, and upper-airway obstruction with respiratory distress.

General Volunteer Instructions:
- Have athlete rest and quickly assess for other injuries.
- Apply cold to the sting site.
- Contact Medical Personnel.

Medical Personnel Instructions:
- Review general volunteer instructions.
- If there are signs of a serious reaction, apply light constrictive band proximal to sting site.
- Remove stinger if it is still present.
- Oral antihistamines (diphenhydramine) will stop the progression of an allergic reaction but does require time to take effect.
- Administer injectible epinephrine if athlete is carrying it and symptoms suggest anaphylaxis.

Additional Medical Director Information:
For athletes exhibiting signs of anaphylaxis, current guidelines recommend immediate evacuation or emergent transport to medical facilities and formal evaluation prior to re-entry. Athletes with only a limited local reaction can

Bites & Stings

resume activity based on the clinical judgment of the medical director.

(Portions of Recommendations Adapted from: Forgey, 94-95)

Bites & Stings

Allergic Reaction

Medical Definition: Immune Hypersensitivity.

Signs & Symptoms: Localized pain, swelling, and redness. A more serious reaction (anaphylaxis) is indicated by the presence of progressive pruritis, hives, or angioedema, and upper-airway obstruction with respiratory distress.

General Volunteer Instructions:
- Have athlete rest and quickly assess for other injuries.
- If there is an inoculation site (bite, sting, etc), apply cold therapy for comfort.
- Contact Medical Personnel.

Medical Personnel Instructions:
- Review general volunteer instructions.
- Oral antihistamines (diphenhydramine) will stop the progression of an allergic reaction but does require time to take effect.
- Administer injectable epinephrine if athlete is carrying it and symptoms suggest anaphylaxis.

Additional Medical Director Information:
Anaphylaxis is a true medical emergency and current guidelines recommend immediate evacuation or emergent transport to medical facilities, and hospital evaluation prior to re-entry. Simple urticaria does not necessitate evacuation if clinical judgment suggests it is limited to the skin and does not involve the airway, gastrointestinal tract, or facial areas. Systemic symptoms should be concerning, and may be a harbinger of impending anaphylaxis.
(Portions of Recommendations Adapted from: Forgey, 95)

7.) MISCELLANEOUS PROBLEMS
Dylan Kellogg & Nathaniel Herr

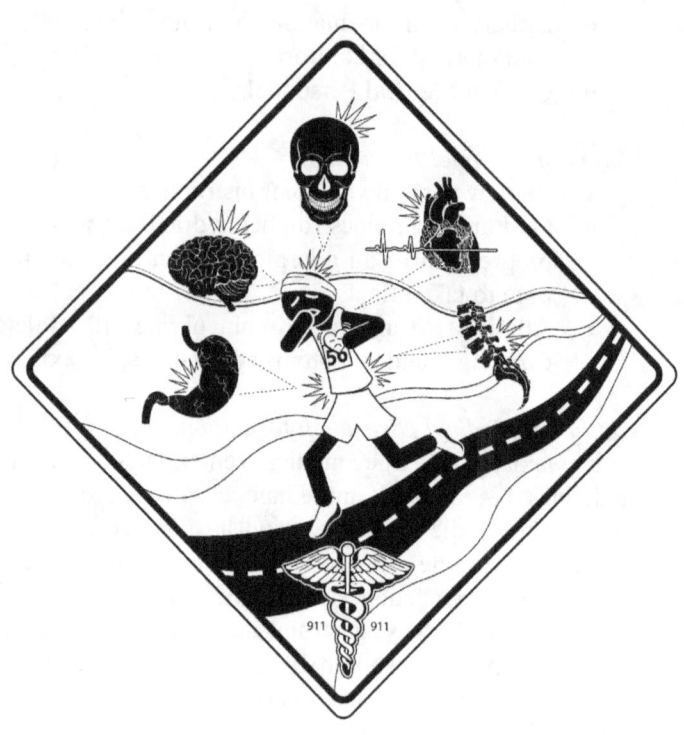

Miscellaneous Problems

Acute Coronary Syndrome

Explanation: Heart Attack.

Medical Definition: Inadequate perfusion of myocardium leading to angina or infarct depending on severity of blockage and degree of tissue hypoxia.

Signs & Symptoms: Chest pain with or without radiation to arm or jaw, nausea, shortness of breath, sweating; decreased BP and increased (or decreased) HR, loss of consciousness.

General Volunteer Instructions:
- Have athlete rest.
- If athlete is awake but not feeling well position them with feet slightly elevated.
- Unless they have an allergy to it, have athlete chew two baby aspirin.
- Contact Medical Personnel.

Medical Personnel Instructions:
- Review general volunteer instructions.
- Provide Basic Life Support for patients who become unresponsive (including utilization of AED per protocol if available).
- Prepare for immediate evacuation or emergent transport to medical facilities.
- If the following medications are available they should be considered as well:
  - 325mg aspirin
  - 300mg clopidogrel
  - 0.4mg SL nitroglycerin if systolic BP is adequate

Miscellaneous Problems

Additional Medical Director Information:
This is a true medical emergency and current guidelines recommend immediate evacuation or emergent transport to medical facilities and formal evaluation prior to re-entry. Although many medications and equipment have been suggested for use in the prehospital environment, current AHA recommendations truly emphasize the use of aspirin, timely transportation to medical facilities, and good compressions for patients who've devolved into cardiac arrest.

(Portions of Recommendations Adapted from: Forgey, 6-12)

Miscellaneous Problems

Concussion / Traumatic Brain Injury

Explanation: Brain injury that may result in a bad headache, altered levels of alertness, or unconsciousness.

Medical Definition: Blow to head that may result in increased intracranial pressure and/or intracranial hemorrhage.

Signs & Symptoms: Headache, feeling "in a fog", emotional lability & personality changes, loss of consciousness, amnesia, irritability, slowed reaction times, drowsiness, visual changes, speech or coordination difficulty, nausea and vomiting, bruising around eyes or ears, fluid in nose/ears. Symptoms might be delayed several hours following injury.

General Volunteer Instructions:
- Contact Medical Personnel immediately.
- Minimize movement (see *Suspected Spinal Injury*).
- If athlete is vomiting, or otherwise having difficulty breathing, position on left side.
- Do not leave athlete alone.

Medical Personnel Instructions:
- Review general volunteer instructions.
- Provide basic life support care as needed
- Assess for possible spinal injury and take indicated precautions.
- If other injuries are present, treat them as indicated in the appropriate section of this text.

Miscellaneous Problems

Additional Medical Director Information:
Unless experienced with concussion management, evaluate using a clinical concussion assessment rule such as SCAT2 (see references). Evaluate athlete over the next few hours, watching for deterioration. If evaluation indicates concussion, it is recommended that athlete not return to race that day. Current guidelines recommend acetaminophen over NSAIDs for pain control. Avoid narcotics. May only return to race after medically cleared. Urgent evacuation or emergent transport to medical facilities are indicated if athlete exhibits signs of increased ICP or skull fracture.

(Portions of Recommendations Adapted from: Forgey, 15-17; McCrory)

Miscellaneous Problems

Suspected Spinal Injury

Explanation: Injury to the spine that should be considered if athlete has suffered a traumatic injury, a significant fall, or trauma to the back or neck.

Medical Definition: Injury to the actual spinal cord or damage to bony spine impinging on cord causing neurologic deficits or risk of developing them.

Signs & Symptoms: Signs of spinal injury include neurologic deficits in extremities; or pain, tenderness, or deformity of the spine.

General Volunteer Instructions:
- Immobilize athlete to prevent worsening of possible spinal injury.
- Contact Medical Personnel.

Medical Personnel Instructions:
- Review general medical instructions.
- Stabilize any life-threatening conditions and treat other injuries as outlined in the appropriate section of this guide.
- If not already done, immobilize athlete.
- If you are unable to clear the spine using clinical decision rules, the athlete must be immobilized and evacuated or transported to medical facilities on a backboard.

Additional Medical Director Information:
Current guidelines recommend evacuation or transport to medical facilities and formal evaluation prior to re-entry.

Miscellaneous Problems

Medical directors may wish to consider immediate evacuation or emergent transport if neurologic deficits are present or if immediate evacuation or transport is indicated by other conditions present. If you are inclined to consider clearing a spine in the field, we recommend using a tool such as the NEXUS criteria (below) or Canadian cervical spine protocol. When applying the NEXUS criteria all of the following must be confirmed or the patient should be immobilized and evacuation or transported as above:

- No pain, tenderness, or deformity of the spine.
- No focal neurologic deficits.
- Normal level of alertness without presence of alcohol/drugs, head injury, or any other state that may result in impairment of consciousness such as AMS.
- No clinically apparent, painful (distracting) injuries.

(Portions of Recommendations Adapted from: Forgey, 18-19; Hoffman)

Miscellaneous Problems

Gastrointestinal Illness

Explanation: Upset stomach.

Medical Definition: Infectious or toxic agent irritating the gastrointestinal system, or visceral pain presenting similarly.

Signs & Symptoms: Nausea, vomiting, diarrhea, constipation, abdominal pain/tenderness.

General Volunteer Instructions:
- Provide fluid with electrolytes (sports drink) if athlete will tolerate.
- Contact Medical Personnel.

Medical Personnel Instructions:
- Review general volunteer instructions.
- Evaluate for, and consider, problems that may necessitate immediate surgical evaluation (e.g. appendicitis)
- Assess athlete for volume status and determine cause of illness if possible
- Assess for red flags: persistent fever, blood per mouth or rectum, persistent vomiting or diarrhea, non-resolving pain, worsening pain, severe tenderness, pertioneal signs, or signs of shock.

Additional Medical Director Information:
Current guidelines recommend immediate evacuation or emergent transport to medical facilities and formal evaluation prior to re-entry if red flags are present, or other acute condition necessitating immediate surgical or medical intervention is suspected. Although empiric antibiotic use is

Miscellaneous Problems

not currently recommended for urban races, an expedition-style race poses unique circumstances in which empiric antibiotic use may be indicated. We recommend reviewing the literature specific to your intended geographic location and local resistance patterns, current CDC recommendations, and athlete's allergy profile to determine the antibiotic of choice.

(Portions of Recommendations Adapted from: Isaac 179-182)

Miscellaneous Problems

Seizure

Medical Definition: Disorganized electrical activity in the brain.

Signs & Symptoms: Can be variable from staring off into space to loss of consciousness with rigidity and/or convulsions.

General Volunteer Instructions:
- Ensure area around seizing athlete is clear.
- Do not restrain or attempt to force something into the mouth.
- Contact Medical Personnel Instructions.

Medical Personnel Instructions:
- Review general volunteer instructions.
- Provide basic life support as needed.
- Place in recovery position and reassure athlete post-seizure.
- Be cognizant that a post-ictal patient may become unknowingly combative or confused. Attempt to protect the athlete from potential sources of harm during this state which may last a few minutes to a several hours.
- Consider possible causes including hypoglycemia, heat stroke, hypoxia, hypotension, electrocution or lightning, toxins, and hyponatremia. Treat any of these as indicated.
- Monitor for recurrent seizure and evacuate or transport.

Miscellaneous Problems

Additional Medical Director Information:
Current guidelines recommend immediate evacuation or emergent transport to medical facilities and formal evaluation prior to re-entry. A patient with a known history of seizure who knowingly accepts the risks of race entry does present a difficult situation for the medical director. These issues should be thoroughly discussed before the race so that properly informed decisions can be made by the athlete and race executives. Possible complications include lowering of the seizure threshold by expected environmental conditions, lability of serum levels of medications, and potentially long periods of time without the presence of witnesses who can summon medical assistance.

(Portions of Recommendations Adapted from: Issac, 63-64)

8.) UNDIFFERENTIATED SYMPTOMS
Jeremy Joslin, MD

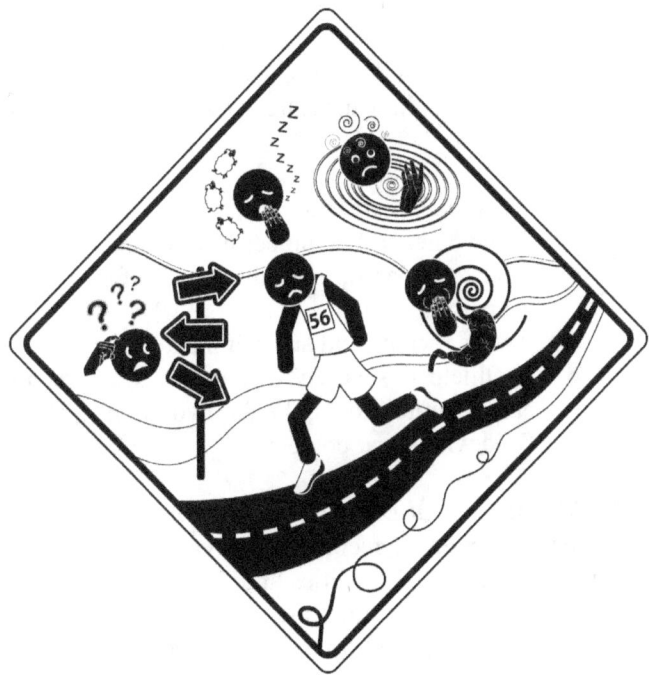

N.B. This section provides a list of commonly encountered symptoms that may be indicative of underlying pathology. While general management guidelines are provided, medical personnel are directed to the chapter appropriate to the underlying condition for additional guidance.

Undifferentiated Symptoms

Confusion

May be seen in dehydration, hyperthermia, hypothermia, heart problem, hyponatremia, stroke, sepsis, renal or liver failure.

General Volunteer Instructions:
- Contact Medical Personnel Instructions.
- Give full strength sports drink if able to swallow normally while sitting up.
- Begin cooling measures if signs of heat illness are present.

Medical Personnel Instructions:
- Review general volunteer instructions.
- Check temperature. If abnormal, refer to appropriate chapter.
- Assess recent fluid and salt intake.
- If athlete is severely dehydrated in appearance and can tolerate fluids, begin hydration with isotonic fluid with sugar content.

Additional Medical Director Information:
Current guidelines recommend evacuation or emergent transport to medical facilities and formal evaluation prior to re-entry. Medical directors may wish to consider immediate evacuation or emergent transport if speech is slurred.

Undifferentiated Symptoms

Abnormal Fatigue

May be seen in hypothermia, hyperthermia, altitude sickness.

General Volunteer Instructions:
- Contact Medical Personnel.

Medical Personnel Instructions:
- If at altitude, descend.
- Check temperature, and if abnormal, refer to appropriate chapter.
- Assess recent fluid and salt intake.
- If athlete is severely dehydrated in appearance and can tolerate fluids, begin hydration with isotonic fluid with sugar content.

Additional Medical Director Information:
Refer to evacuation and transport guidelines as per underlying problem. Requirements for re-entry as per underlying problem.

Undifferentiated Symptoms

Dizziness

Can be seen in altitude sickness, hyperthermia.

General Volunteer Instructions:
- Contact Medical Personnel.

Medical Personnel Instructions:
- If at altitude, descend.
- Check temperature, and if abnormal, refer to appropriate chapter.
- Assess recent fluid and salt intake.
- If athlete is severely dehydrated in appearance and can tolerate fluids, begin hydration with isotonic fluid with sugar content.

Additional Medical Director Information:
Refer to evacuation and transport guidelines as per underlying problem. Requirements for re-entry as per underlying problem.

Undifferentiated Symptoms

Vomiting

Can be seen in altitude sickness, drowning, hyperthermia, traumatic brain injury, gastrointestinal illness, seizure.

General Volunteer Instructions:
- Contact Medical Personnel.
- May offer sips of fluids if athlete is fully conscious.

Medical Personnel Instructions:
- Review general volunteer instructions.
- Assess for traumatic brain injury.
- If at altitude, descend.
- Check temperature, and if abnormal, refer to appropriate chapter.
- Assess recent fluid and salt intake.
- If athlete is severely dehydrated in appearance and can tolerate fluids, begin hydration with isotonic fluid with sugar content.
- **Oral ondansetron is recommended to assist athlete in orally hydrating**.
- Recent literature suggests that empiric use of intravenous fluids is not needed in most cases of race-induced vomiting that has been carefully attributed to heat intolerance.

Additional Medical Director Information:
Current guidelines recommend immediate evacuation or emergent transport and formal evaluation for severe, continuous vomiting, or vomiting due to an underlying serious problem. Isolated vomiting does not generally warrant evacuation, but it is prudent for all episodes of

Undifferentiated Symptoms

vomiting to be evaluated and if race re-entry is desired, cleared by medical director prior to re-entry.

(Portions of Recommendations Adapted from: Noakes)

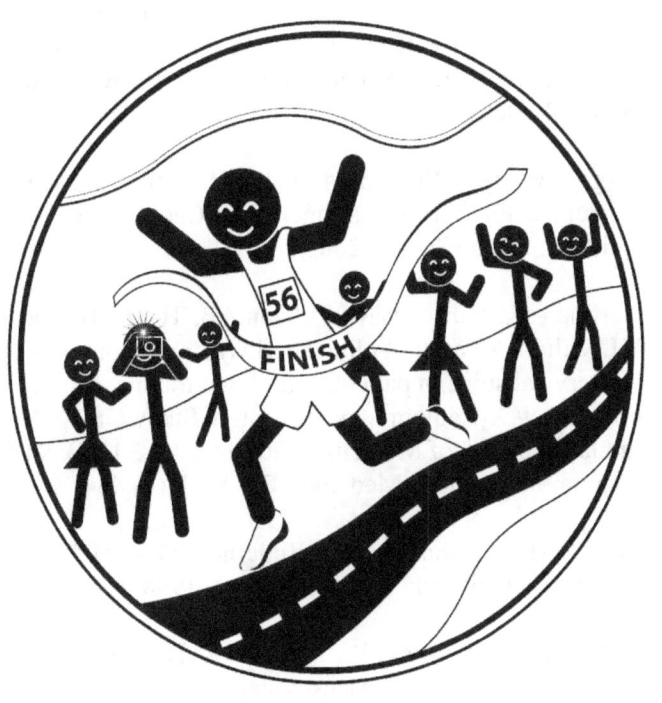

References

Carline JD, Lentz MJ, Macdonald SC. Mountaineering Fist Aid: A Guide to Accident Response and First Aid Care. 5th ed. Seattle: The Mountaineers Books, 2004.

Castellani JW, Young AJ, Ducharme MB, Giesbrecht GG, Glickman E, Sallis RE. Prevention of cold injuries during exercise. Medicine & Science in Sports & Exercise. 2006; 38: 2012-2029.

Forgey WM, ed. Wilderness Medical Society: Practice Guidelines for Wilderness Emergency Care. 5th ed. Guilford: FalconGuides, 2006.

Hoffman JR, Mower WR, Wolfson AB, Todd KH, Zucker MI. Validity of a set of clinical criteria to rule out injury to the cervical spine in patients with blunt trauma. National Emergency X-Radiography Utilization Study Group. New England Journal of Medicine. 2000 July 13; 343(2): 94-99. Erratum in: N Engl J Med 2001 Feb 8;344(6):464.

Isaac J. The Outward Bound Wilderness First-Aid Handbook. Guilford: The Lyons Press, 1998.

McCrory P, Meeuwisse W, Johnston K, Dvorak J, Aubry M, Molloy M, Cantu R. Consensus statement on concussion in sport - the 3rd international conference on concussion in sport held in Zurich, November 2008. 2009; 1(5): 406-420.

Micheli LJ, ed. Encyclopedia of Sports Medicine. 1st ed. Sage Publications Inc., 2011.

Noakes T. Fluid replacement during marathon running. Clinical Journal of Sports Medicine. 2003; 13: 309-318.

References

Rogers IR, Hew-Butler, T. Exercise-associated hyponatremia: overzealous fluid consumption. Wilderness and Environmental Medicine. 2009; 20: 139-143.

Seto CK, Way D, O'Connor N. Environmental Illness in Athletes. Clinics in Sports Medicine. 2005; 24: 695-718.

Trojian TH, McKeag, DB. Ankle Sprains: Expedient Assessment and Management. The Physician and Sportsmedicine. 1998; 26(10): 106-116.